<u>Recipes to Rave About</u>:
Outrageously Delicious Main Dishes for People on the RAVE Diet*

by Laurie J. Mauro

Dedicated with love, to my darling daughter Ali, who was both my inspiration for creating this cookbook and my taste-tester.

TABLE OF CONTENTS

A. Explanation of RAVE Diet*

B. Recipes

C. Create Your Own Recipes, Using UnCommon Substitutions for Ingredients
Avoided on RAVE Diet

Recipes to Rave About:
Outrageously Delicious Main Dishes
for People on the RAVE Diet*

RAVE is an acronym which stands for: No Refined foods, No Animal foods, No Vegetable oils, and No Exceptions and Exercise.

The RAVE Diet was developed by Mike Anderson, after extensive research into the relationship between diet and disease. He found that many common illnesses, such as heart disease, diabetes and cancers can be halted and reversed by following some basic rules for eating. Citing many studies done by major medical institutions and well-known nutritionists and doctors, he came to the conclusion that a healthy vegan diet is crucial to avoiding disease. The RAVE diet, which goes even beyond vegan guidelines, is endorsed by the Cleveland Clinic Foundation and is being used in wellness centers throughout the world.

This cookbook was created as a loving answer to my own daughter's health concerns. She was convinced that the RAVE diet would provide a cure for her, and so I set out to find substitutions for ingredients we could no longer use in our family recipes. My goal was to keep meals delicious while staying within the RAVE dictates. After much experimentation and research, success came for both of us! After a year and a half, Ali is completely healthy and I am sharing some of the recipes that have kept her happily on the diet. She is still eating RAVE, and loving it!

The "Substitutions" page alone is worth many times the cost of this cookbook. These substitutions can be used to create your own recipes, based on the tried and true meals your family already enjoys. I've found the less your food tastes *different* while you're transitioning, the more likely you'll be able to make this RAVE lifestyle change permanent, and keep you and your family healthy way into the future.

Stay tuned for Volume 2, with some great dessert recipes! Yes, desserts!

Email ravedietrecipes@gmail.com to be included on our mailing list for updates!

*RAVE Diet was developed by Mike Anderson, author of "The RAVE Diet and Lifestyle."

RECIPES

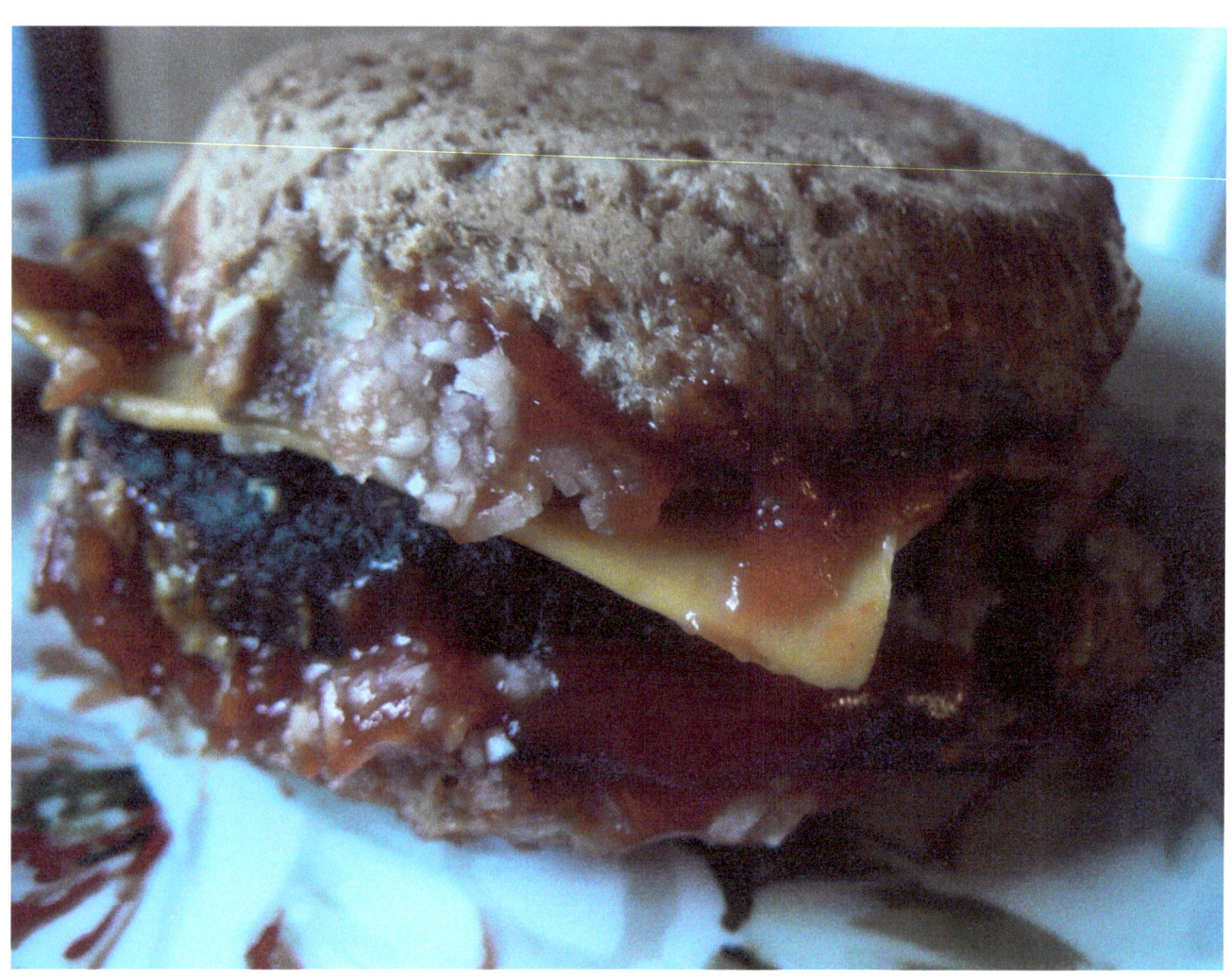

MICKEY V'S CHEESEBURGER

Ingredients:

1 teaspoon dried onion flakes
4 teaspoons boiling water
1 vegan "hamburger" (Use the BLACK BEAN VEGGIE BURGER recipe in this cookbook)
1 Ezekiel hamburger bun
2 tablespoons ketchup
1 teaspoon mustard
1 dill pickle slice
1 slice Go Veggie vegan American cheese

Directions:

1. Pour boiling water over the dried onion flakes and let stand until completely hydrated.

2. Prepare BLACK BEAN VEGGIE BURGER, according to recipe in book.

3. Heat bun on the grill or by browning in a frying pan.

4. Spread half of the ketchup on bottom half of bun, then half the mustard and onions.

5. Spread the other half on the top of the bun and add pickle slice.

6. Place burger on bottom half, cover with "cheese."

7. Place top half of bun on top and enjoy!

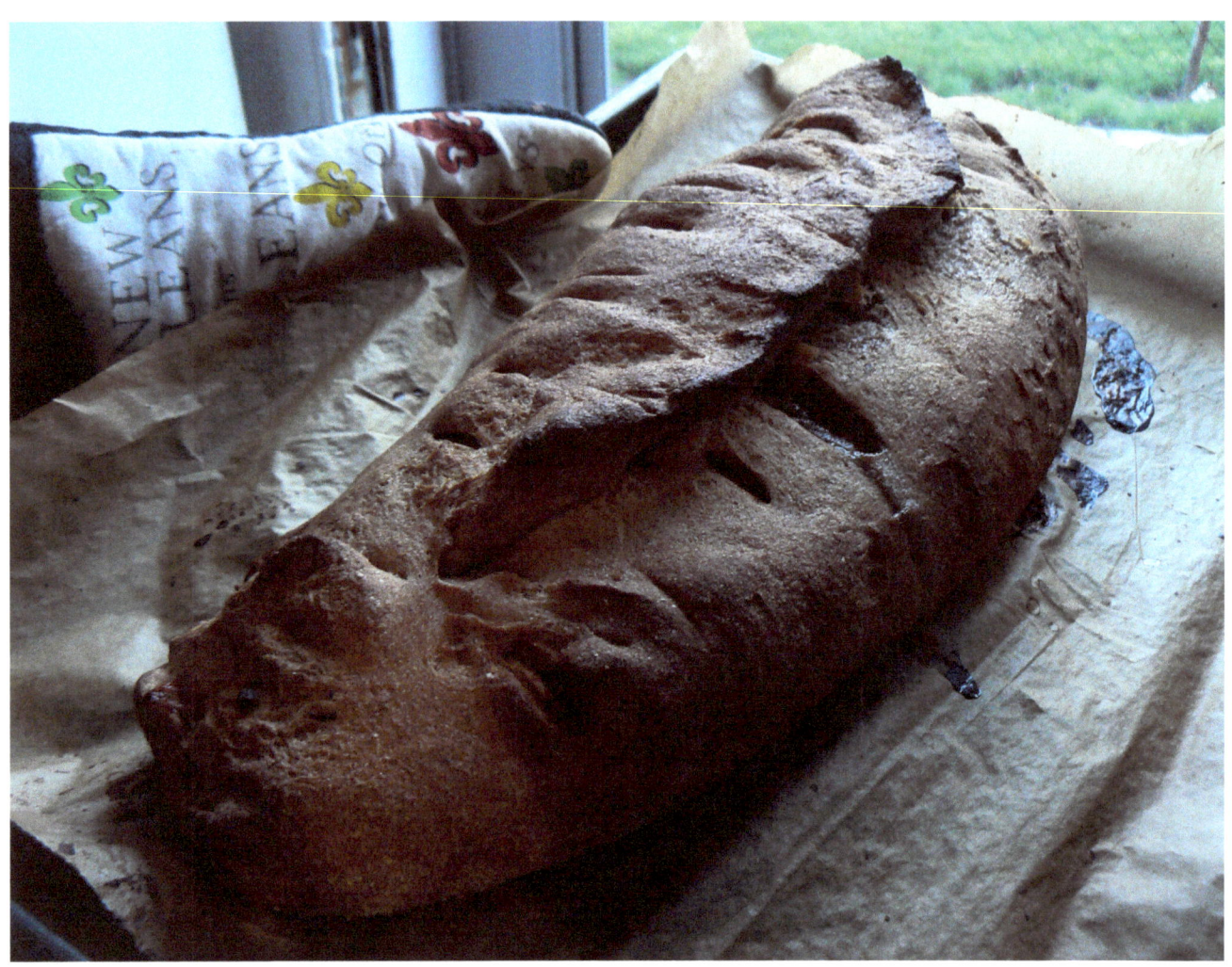

CALZONE

Ingredients:
PASTRY DOUGH:

1 cup water

¼ cup almond milk

1 teaspoon sea salt

1 tablespoon agave

1 teaspoon flax seed meal

3 cups whole wheat bread flour

2 teaspoons active dry yeast

FILLING:

1 cup pasta sauce

¾ cup chopped zucchini

¾ cup grated potato

1 teaspoon fennel

1 teaspoon flax seed meal, mixed with ¼ cup water
to brush the top of calzone before baking

Parchment paper

Directions:

1. Preheat oven to 350 degrees.
2. Place water, almond milk, salt, agave, one teaspoon flax seed meal, bread flour and yeast in bread machine. Select dough cycle.
3. After cycle ends, roll out dough on lightly floured surface, shaping into a 16 x10 inch rectangle. Transfer to cookie sheet, lined with parchment paper.
4. In a bowl, mix together zucchini, potato and fennel.
5. Spoon pasta sauce in a stip down the center of dough lengthwise. Add zucchini/potato mixture.
6. Make diagonal cuts 1-1/2 inches apart down both sides of dough, cutting to ½ inches of the filling.
7. Fold both sides of dough over the filled center and seal with flax seed/water mixture, brushing top lightly with it as well.
8. Bake for 35 to 40 minutes. Watch and cover with aluminum foil, if crust starts to brown too fast.

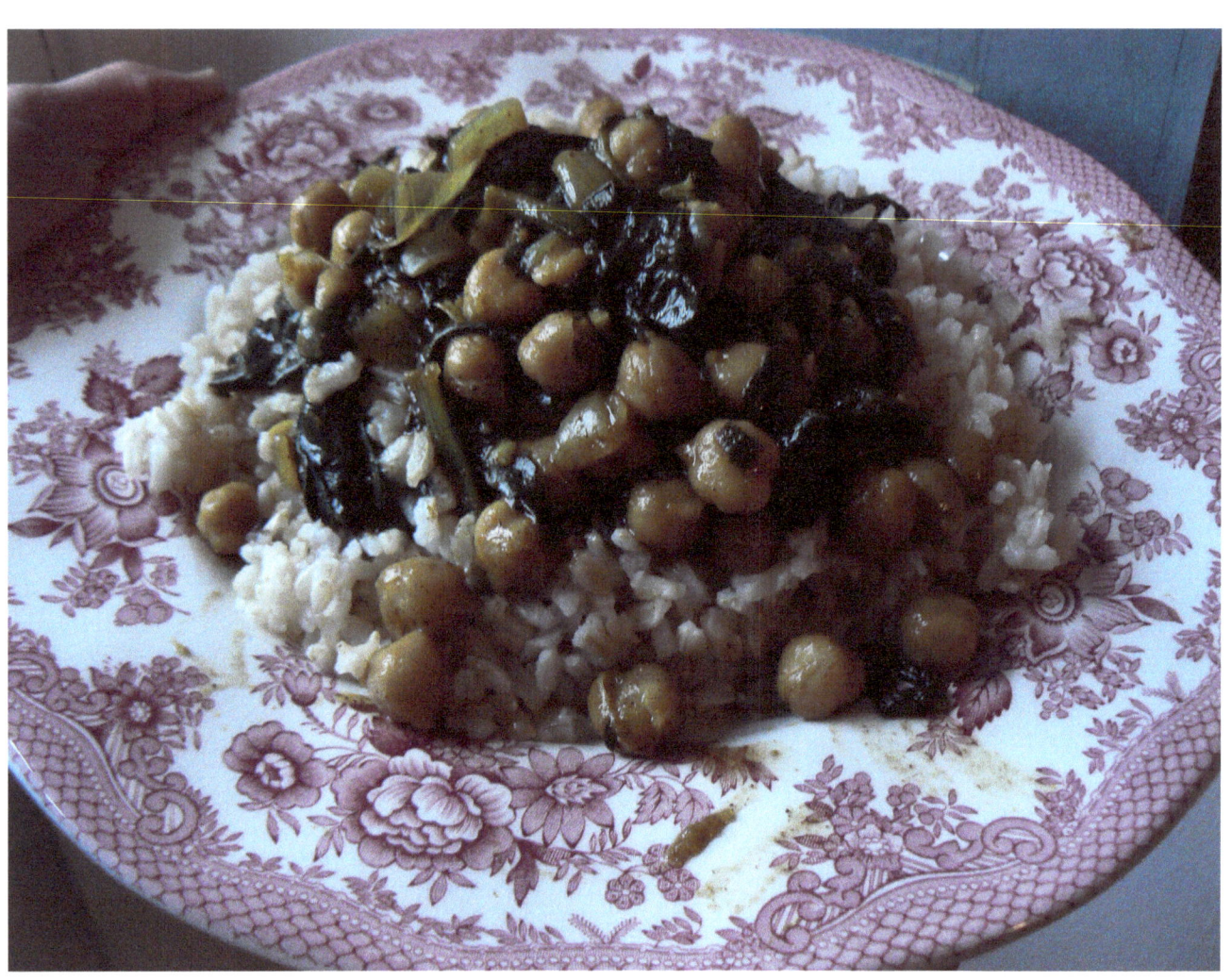

CHANA SAAG

Ingredients:

1- 16oz can chickpeas w/water
1 small onion, diced
3 cloves garlic, minced
1/8 cup water
2 tbs. Lemon juice
½ tsp curry powder
½ tsp coriander powder
½ tsp cumin
½ tsp garam masala
1 bunch of spinach, washed

Directions:

1. In a large skillet, heat water and sautee onion and garlic in hot liquid, until onion is translucent and the garlic aromatic.

2. Add chickpeas, along with its water. Add all lemon juice and all spices; simmer, stirring occasionally for 15 minutes.

3. Reduce heat. Add spinach and cover. Cook for just a few minutes, until spinach is wilted.

Serve over brown rice!

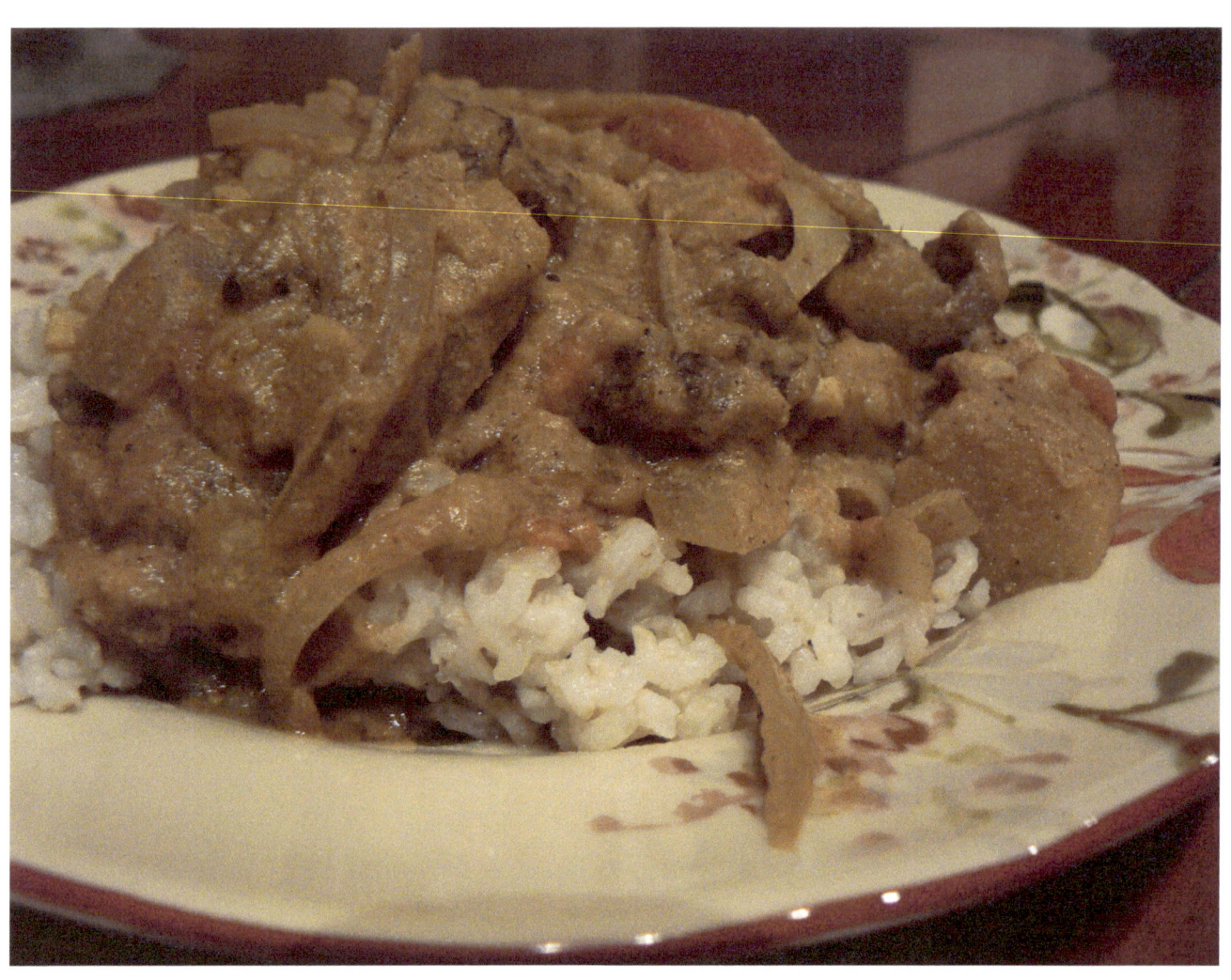

EGGPLANT CURRY

Ingredients:

1 large eggplant
1 cup water, divided
1 medium onion, thinly sliced
1 tablespoon fresh grated ginger
1 tablespoon cumin
1 tablespoon curry powder
1 teaspoon garlic powder
1 tomato, diced
4 tablespoons tahini paste (mix with two large cloves garlic, 2 tablespoons lemon juice
    and add enough water to make ½ cup)
1 teaspoon sea salt
¼ cup fresh cilantro, for garnish

Directions:

1. Preheat oven to 450 degrees F
2. Place eggplant on a baking sheet and bake 20-30 minutes, until tender. Remove from oven, cool, peel and then chop.
3. Heat ½ cup water in a saucepan over medium heat, and mix in onion and ginger. Cook until onion is tender, and then add the cumin and curry powder.
4. Stir until water is all evaporated, to release the full flavor of the spices.
5. Add the rest of the water, garlic powder, tomato, and tahini mixture.
6. Mix in eggplant and sea salt. Cover and simmer about 10 minutes.
7. Garnish with cilantro and serve!

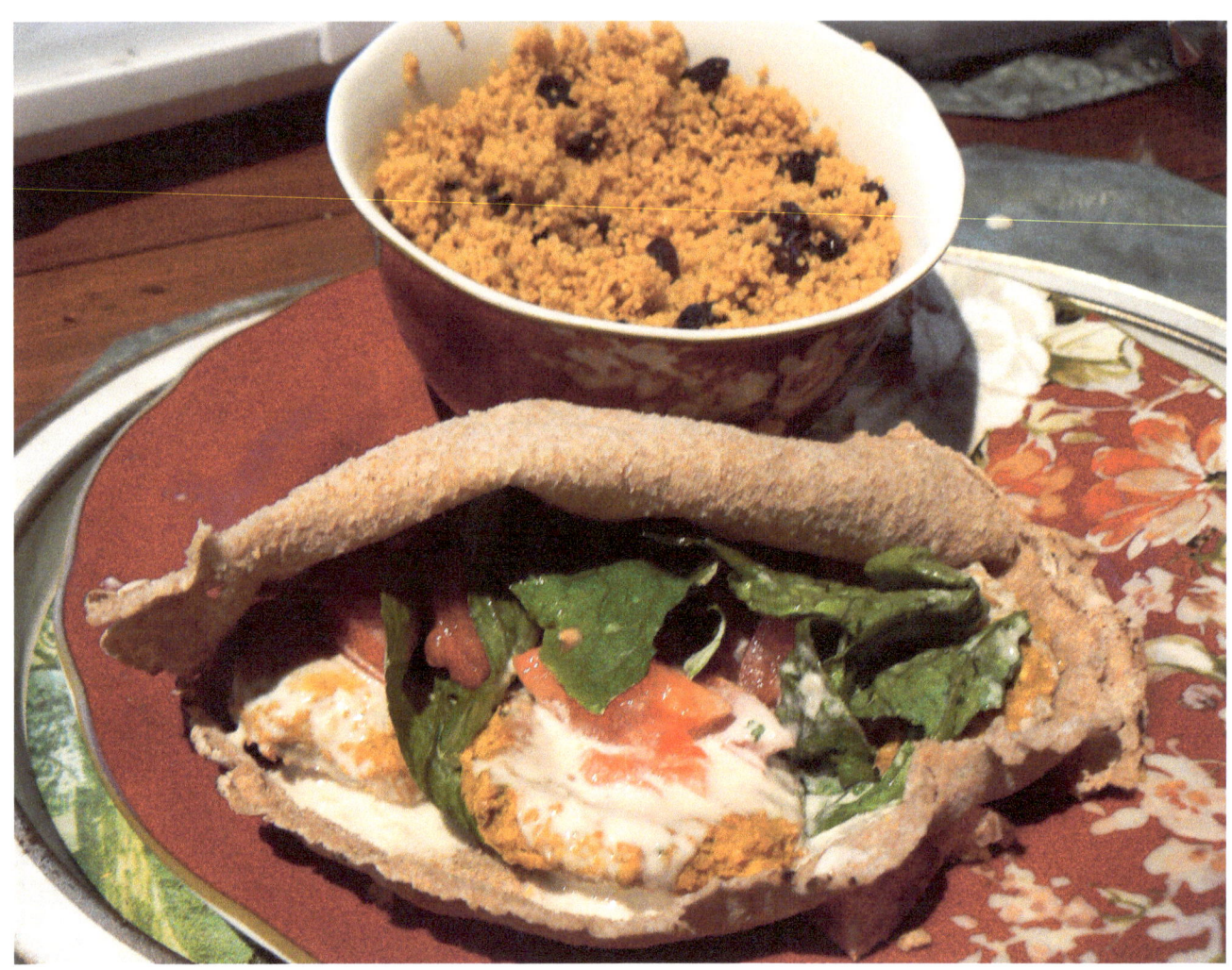

FELAFELS WITH TAHINI SAUCE

Ingredients:

1 can chickpeas, drained
1 onion, chopped finely
½ cup fresh parsley
2 cloves garlic, chopped
1 tsp. Flaxseed powder,
     mixed w/ ¼ cup water
2 tsp. ground cumin
1 tsp. ground coriander
1 tsp. sea salt

1/8 tsp. ground pepper
1 pinch cayenne pepper
1 tsp. lemon juice
1 tsp. baking powder
1 Tbs. applesauce
1 cup dry bread crumbs,
     made from Ezekiel bread
     in food processor
Parchment paper

1. Whisk flaxseed powder and water together in a large bowl.
Mash chickpeas with a fork and add to bowl, along with the rest of the ingredients. Let sit for 15 minutes, and line a cookie sheet with parchment paper. (The parchment paper will add a crispness to the felafel patties, similar to frying.)

2. Preheat oven to 375 degrees.

3. Form 2-inch patties by making balls and flattening them with a fork after they are placed on the parchment paper.

4. Place in 375-degree oven and cook until the bottom side shows signs of crispness, and then turn. Bake for five more minutes. The middle of patties should still be somewhat soft.

Enjoy, with whole wheat pitas, chopped salad and tahini sauce!

TAHINI SAUCE:

In food processor, blend together until slightly creamy (slowly adding water, if necessary):

¼ cup JOYVAr Sesame Tahini
¼ cup water
2 tablespoons lemon juice
1/8 teaspoon sea salt
2 cloves garlic

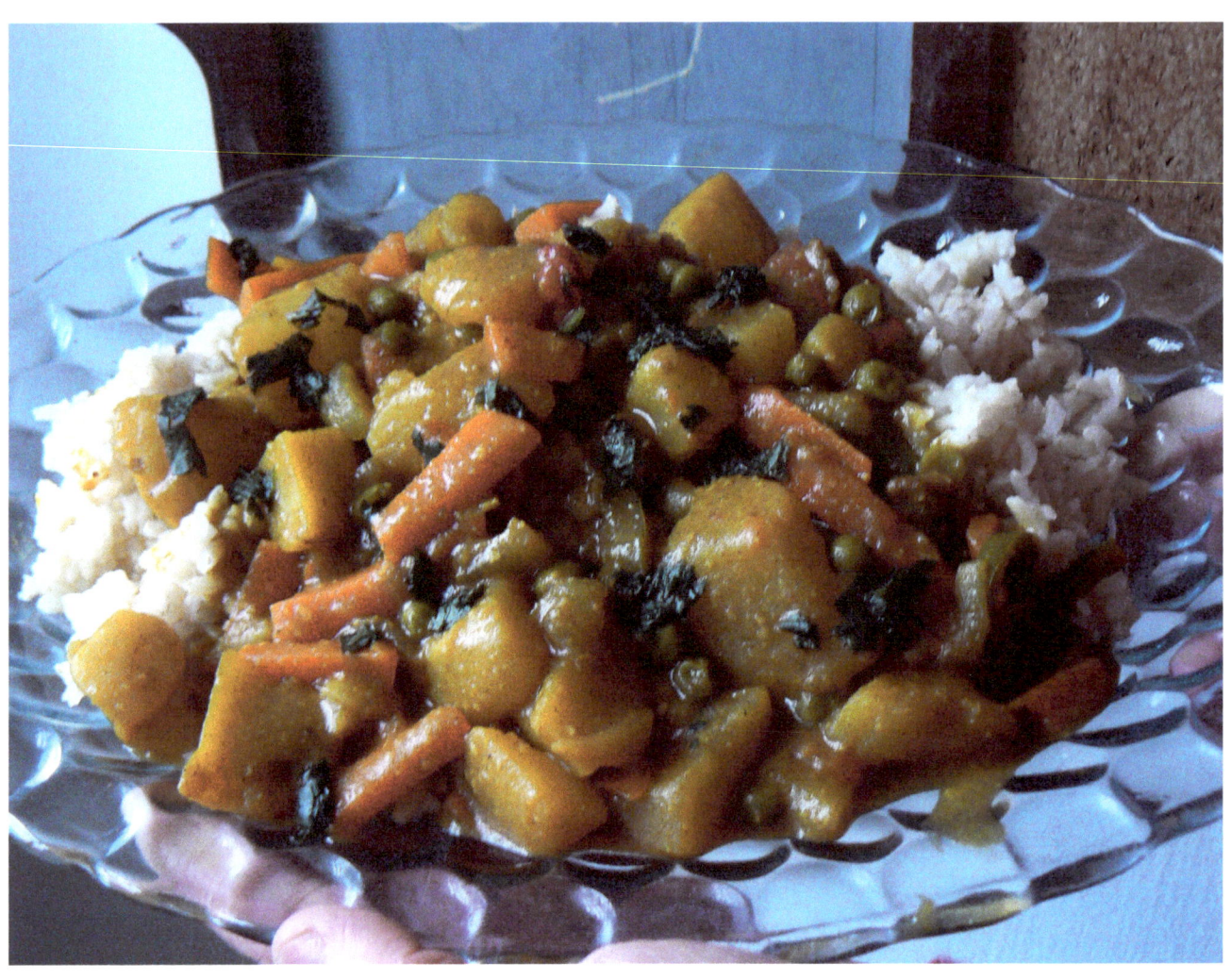

SLOW COOKER INDIAN COCONUT VEGETARIAN CURRY

Ingredients:

5 Russet potatoes, peeled and cut into 1" cubes
¼ cup curry powder
1 tsp. Garam masala
2 tablespoons corn starch
1 tsp. chili powder
1/8 tsp cayenne pepper
1 large green bell pepper, cut into strips
1 large red bell pepper, cut into strips
1 medium onion
1 ½ cups matchstick-cut carrots
1 cup green peas
1- 14 oz can coconut milk
1 cup water
½ tsp garlic powder
¼ tsp black pepper
½ tsp sea salt
¼ cup chopped fresh cilantro

Directions:

1. Place the potatoes in the bottom of the slow cooker.
2. Mix the curry powder, garam masala, cornstarch, chili powder, cayenne together in a small bowl. Sprinkle over potatoes, and stir to coat evenly.
3. Add green and red pepper, onion, carrots and peas , then water and coconut milk, garlic powder, black pepper and salt.
4. Stir to combine.
5. Cook on LOW for 8 hours.
6. Garnish with fresh cilantro before serving.

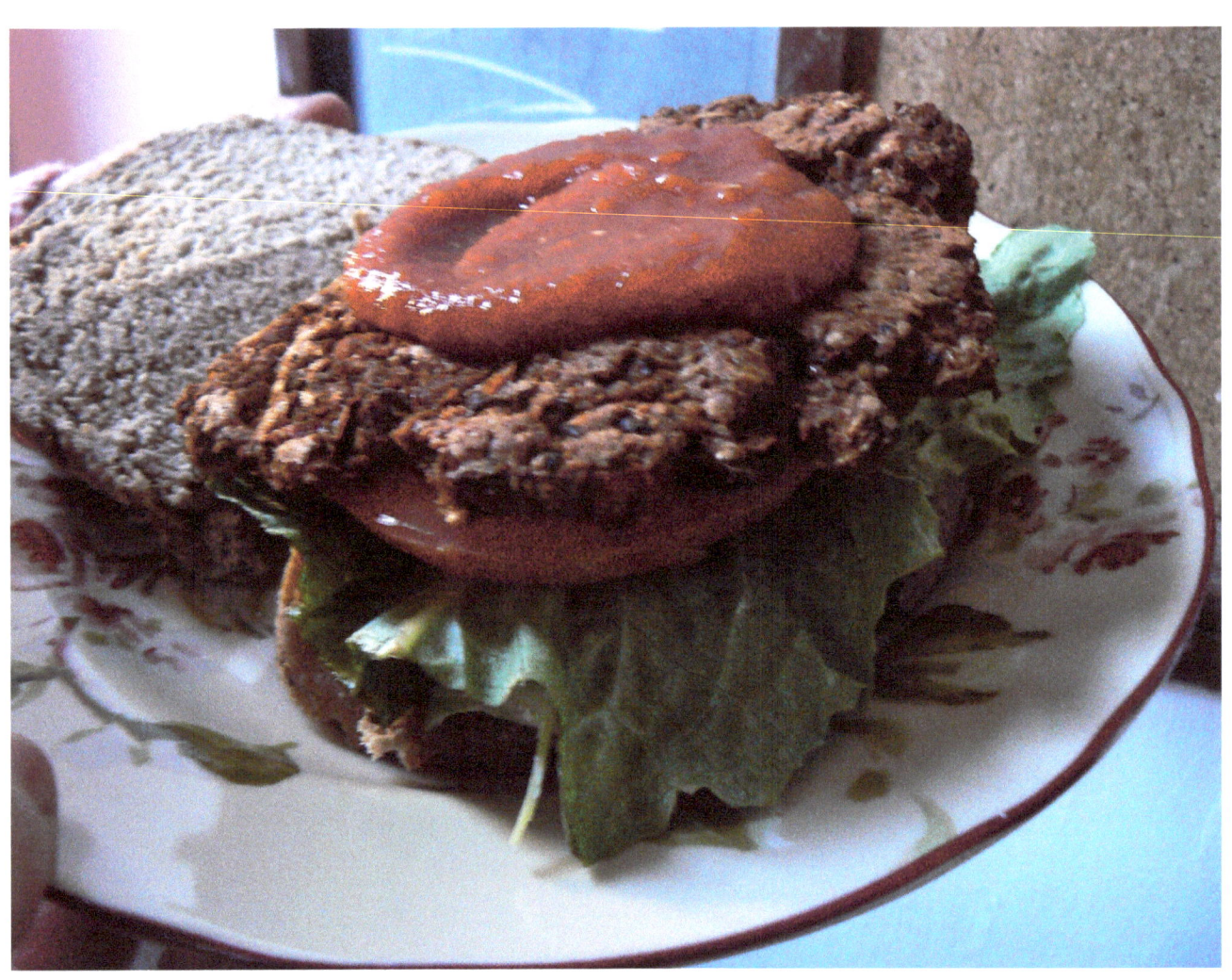

BLACK BEAN VEGGIE BURGERS

Ingredients:

1- 16 oz. Can black beans, drained and rinsed
½ red bell pepper, cut into chunks
½ onion, cut into wedges
4 cloves peeled garlic
1 tablespoon flaxseed powder, dissolved in 3 tablespoons water
(mix until well blended and has the consistency of egg)
1 teaspoon chili powder
1 tablespoon ground cumin
1 teaspoon salsa
3/4 cup bread crumbs, made from Ezekiel bread in food processor

Directions:

1. Preheat oven to 375 degrees. Line a cookie sheet with parchment paper.
2. Place beans, red pepper, onion and cloves in food processor on low, until well mixed and beans are like mashed.
3. In a small bowl, mix together flaxseed mixture, chili powder and cumin.
4. Add spice mixture to beans, along with salsa and bread crumbs. Mix well.
5. Form into four patties and flatten to ½ inch on parchment paper.
6. Bake approximately 15 minutes on each side, until both sides are crispy and insides are firm.
7. Serve on Ezekiel bread, with lettuce, tomato and homemade ketchup!

KETCHUP:
2 tablespoons tomato paste
1 teaspoon apple cider vinegar
¼ teaspoon onion powder
agave to taste

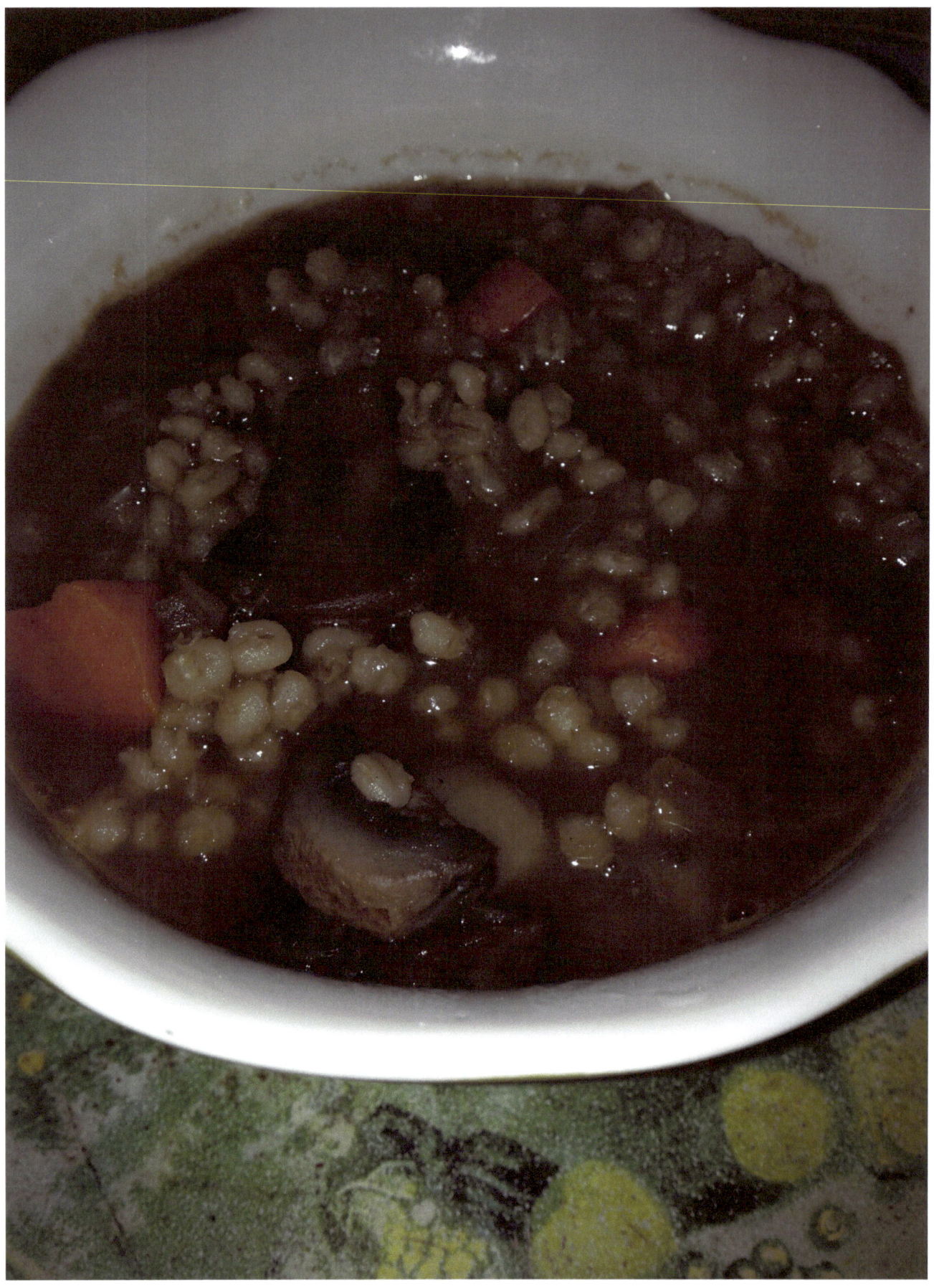

MUSHROOM BARLEY SOUP

Ingredients:

1 cup barley
4 cups water, divided
2 onions, quartered and sliced thin
1 carrot, sliced thin
2 stalks celery, sliced thin
2-8 oz. packages sliced mushrooms
5 cups vegetable broth
½ teaspoon salt
¼ teaspoon ground black pepper

Directions:

1. Bring the barley and 3 cups of the water to a boil, lower the heat to simmer for about 30 minutes or until tender. Set aside.
2. Heat the remaining cup of water in a soup pot and add onions, carrot and celery. Cook about 10 minutes and then add mushrooms, heating 5-10 minutes more.
3. Add vegetable broth and when soup is simmering, lower heat to medium-low. Simmer for 15 minutes more, and then stir in barley.
4. Salt and pepper before serving.

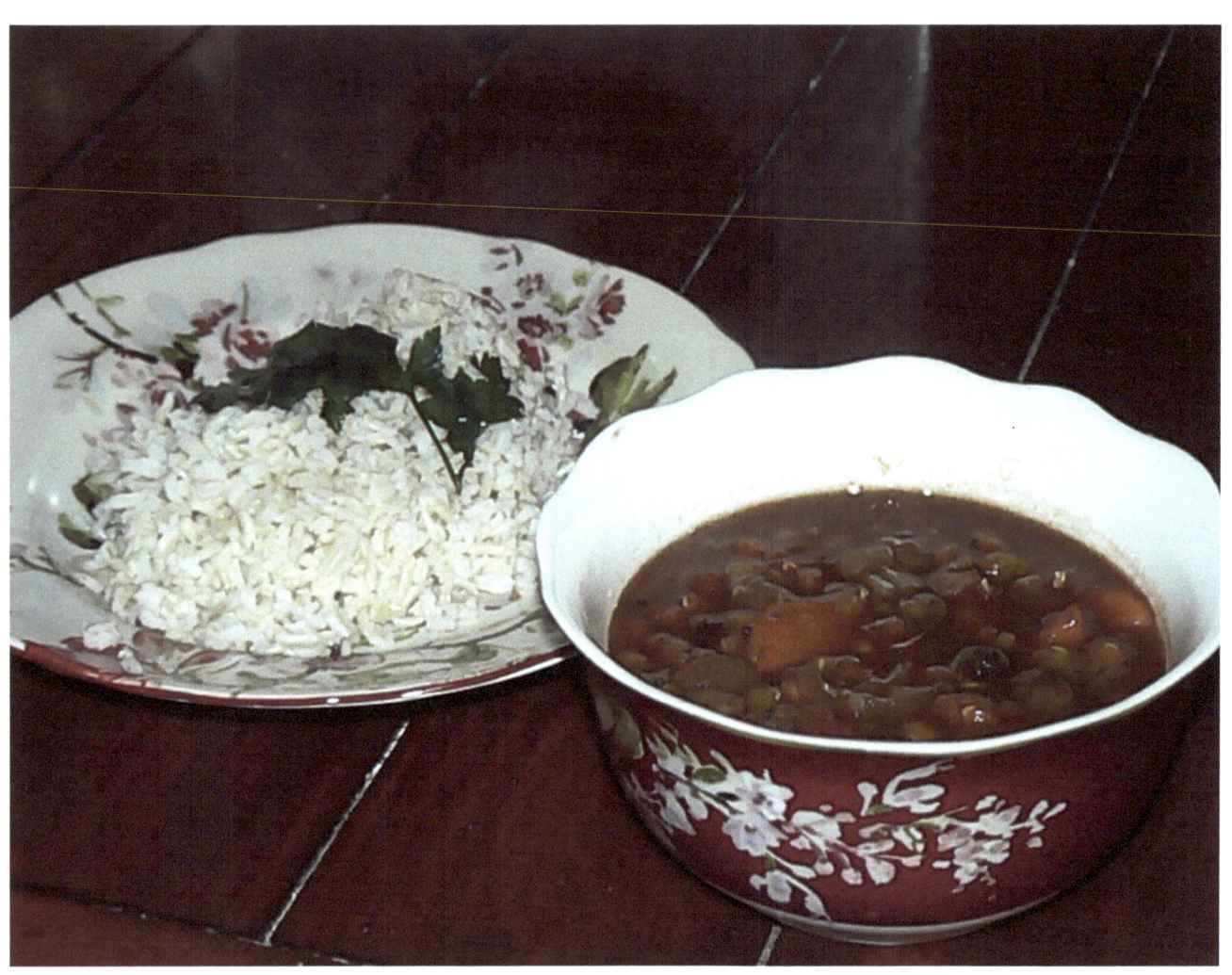

SLOW COOKER LENTIL SOUP

Ingredients:

½ cup lentils, rinsed
½ cup chopped celery
½ cup chopped carrots
½ cup chopped onion
3 cloves garlic minced
3 cups water
1 – 1 lb can diced tomatoes
1 small can tomato sauce
½ tsp sea salt
¼ tsp ground black pepper
2 tsps. cumin
½ tsp tumeric
1/8 tsp ground cloves
1/4 tsp. cinnamon
handful of raisins

Directions:

1. Place all ingredients in the slow cooker
2. Mix and cook on low for 8 hrs.

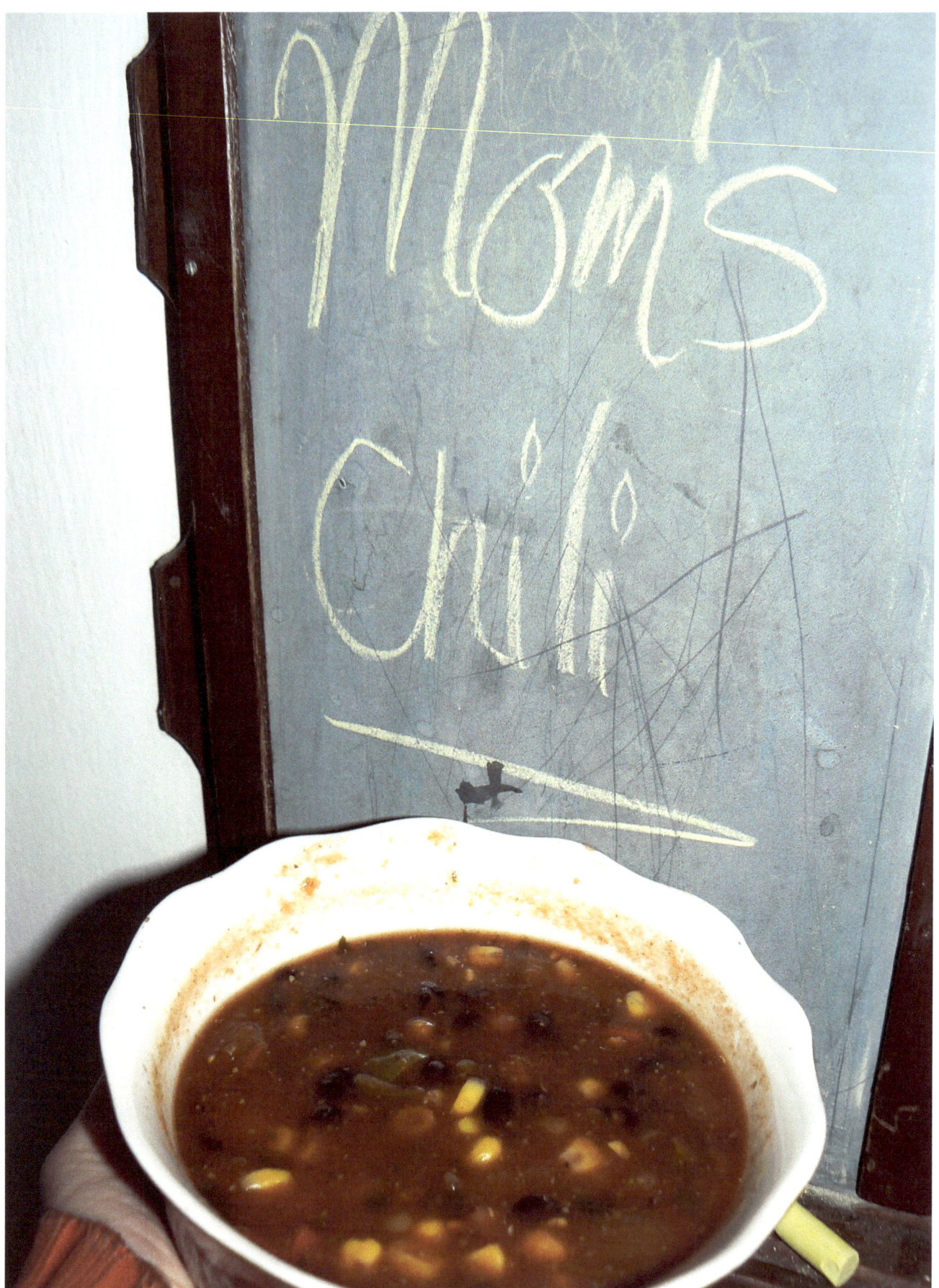

VEGETARIAN CHILI IN SLOW COOKER

Ingredients:

2 cups mushrooms, chopped
1 medium onion, chopped
1 cup chopped carrot
¾ cup chopped green pepper
¼ cup chopped celery
4 cloves garlic, minced
1 tbs. Chili powder
1 tbs. Ground cumin
1 tsp sea salt
½ tsp ground black pepper
¾ tsp dried basil
¾ tsp dried oregano
1 – 28 oz can whole peeled tomatoes, with juice
3 cups beans (black, pinto, white beans in any combination)
½ can tomato paste
¼ cup red wine
¼ tsp cayenne
2 cups water

Directions:

1. Put all ingredients in the slow cooker.
2. Cook on LOW for 5-6 hours

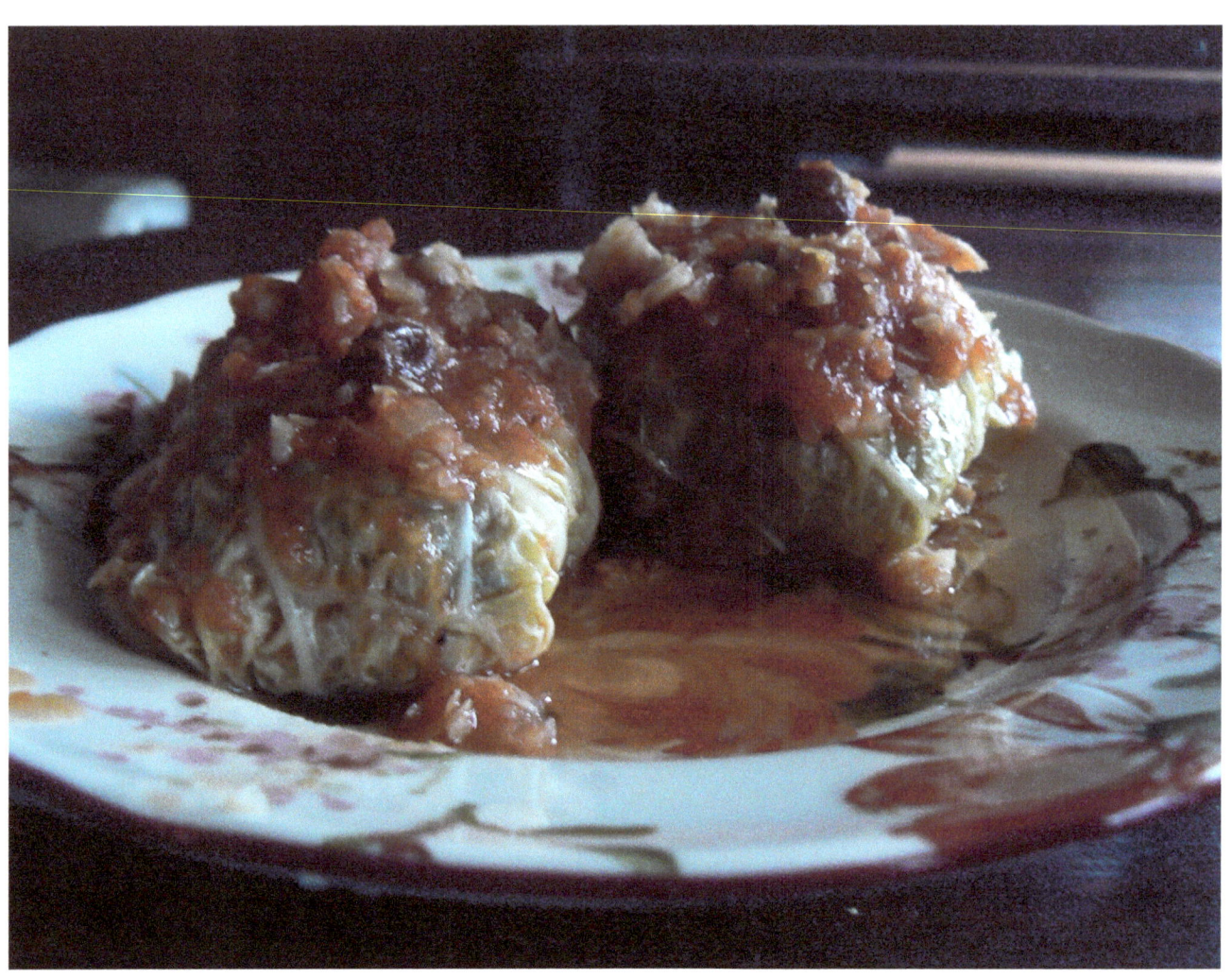

STUFFED CABBAGE

Ingredients:

SAUCE:
1 medium onion, chopped
pinch of baking soda
4 cloves garlic, minced
2- 28 oz cans whole tomatoes,
    pureed in blender
2 tablespoons tomato paste
1 teaspoon salt
¼ teaspoon black pepper
1 tablespoon lemon juice
1 tablespoon agave

FILLING:
3 cups cooked lentils
1 cup cooked brown rice
1 med. onion, chopped
2 cloves garlic, minced
1/8 cup fresh parsley, chopped
2 Tbs. lemon juice
1 tsp. paprika
½ tsp. black pepper
½ tsp. sea salt
¼ tsp. allspice

CABBAGE AND ADDITIONS:
1 head cabbage
1 carrot, peeled and cut into thin circles (added to pot just before cooking)

Directions:
1. Heat ¼ cup water in saucepan; add onions and pinch of baking soda. Cook until the onions are translucent (about 5 minutes), then add garlic for another minute. Add all remaining sauce ingredients, except the raisins. Simmer on low, with cover.
2. Fill a deep pot with enough water to cover whole cabbage and bring to a boil. Remove the core, as much as possible, from the cabbage and place core side up into the boiling water. Boil until leaves soften and begin to come free of the cabbage head. Strain cabbage in a colander, under cold water. Remove at least a dozen leaves from the head, to be filled. Cut up remaining cabbage and add to simmering sauce with raisins.
3. Prepare filling, adding all ingredients and mixing well. Pour one half of the sauce on the bottom of a large pan or dutch oven.
4. Stem side toward you, fill the bottom of each leaf with about 1/3 cup of the filling —rolling upwards and then folding the sides in. Place each cabbage roll in the sauce in a single layer, until all the filling is used. Pour the other half of the sauce on top of rolls, add carrots and simmer on very low setting, covered, until cabbage is tender, about two hours.

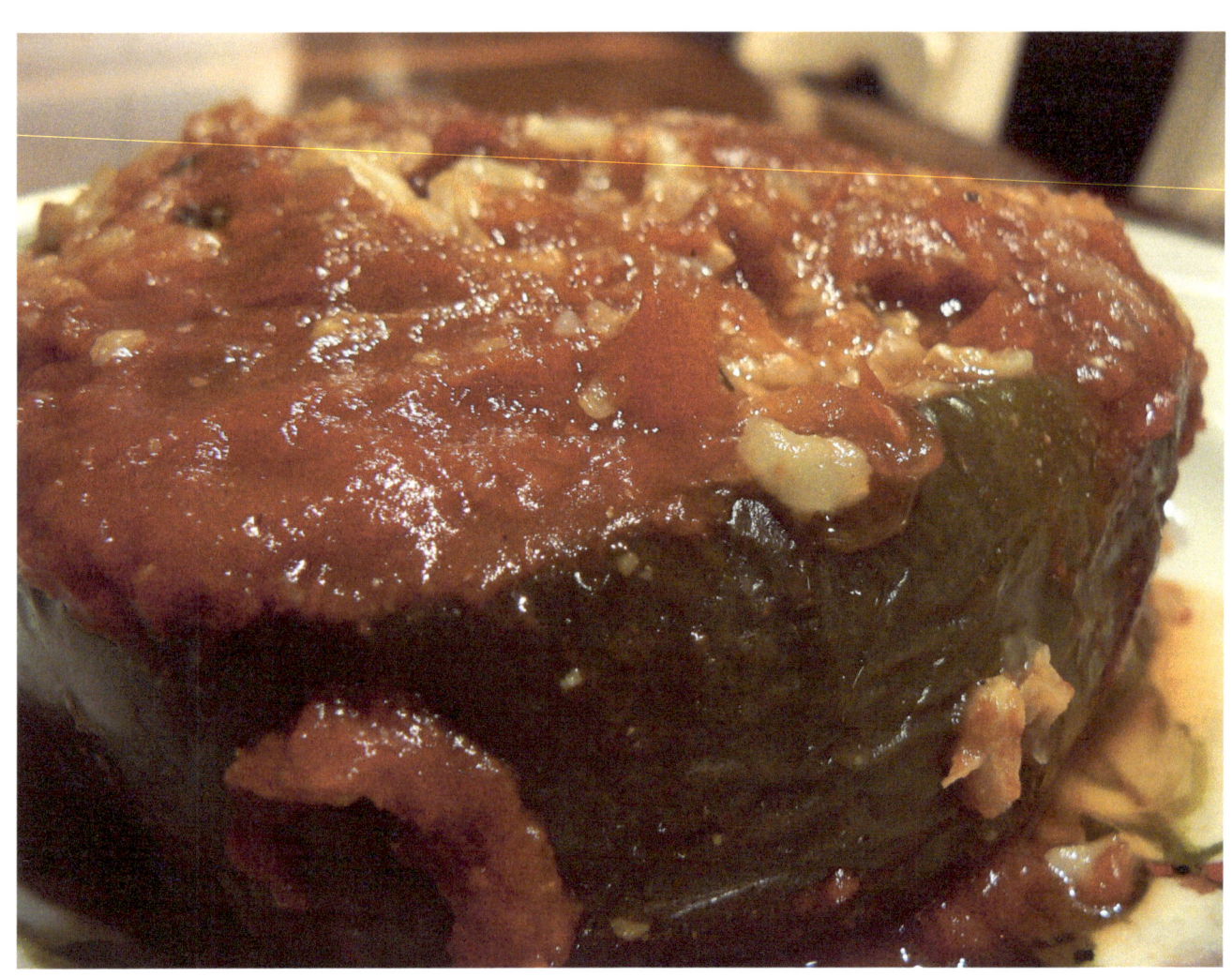

STUFFED PEPPERS

Ingredients:
SAUCE:
2 cups tomato sauce
½ onion, chopped
1 cup vegetable broth
1 tablespoon balsamic vinegar
1/8 teaspoon cayenne pepper

FILLING:
1 cup uncooked brown rice
2 cups water
½ onion
2 – 1 lb cans chick peas, drained and mashed
1- 10oz can diced tomatoes
¼ cup fresh Italian parsley
4 cloves garlic, minced
2 teaspoons sea salt
½ teaspoon ground black pepper
1/8 teaspoon cayenne pepper
1 tablespoon fennel
¼ cup Bragg Nutritional Yeast Seasoning

4 large green peppers, halved and seeded
Additional Bragg Nutritional Yeast Seasoning to sprinkle on top.

Directions:
1. Cook one cup rice in two cups water until tender and set aside.
2. Preheat oven to 375 degrees.
3. Chop one onion and saute in ½ cup water for five minutes, divide in half—half goes in bowl for filling, the other half stays in pan. Add sauce ingredients to onion and heat for a few minutes.
4. Pour sauce into 9 x 12 baking pan.
5. Place pepper halves into baking pan on top of sauce.
6. Mix all the ingredients for filling together in a large bowl, and fill the pepper halves.
7. Sprinkle additional Bragg Nutritional Yeast over top of peppers.
8. Cover tightly with aluminum foil and bake in oven for 45 minutes. Then remove foil and bake an additional 25 minutes, until peppers are tender and filling hot.
9. Spoon sauce from pan over peppers to serve.

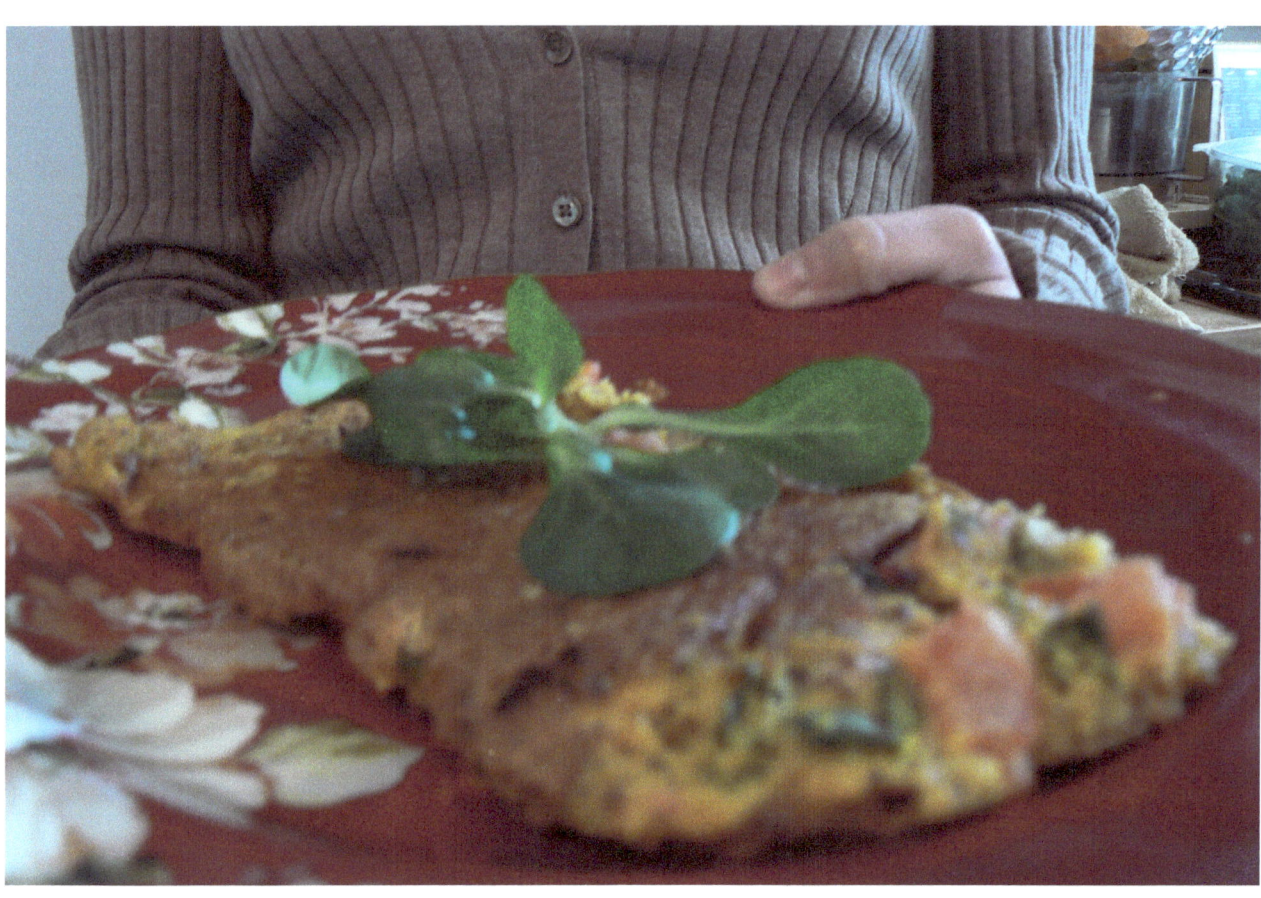

VEGAN OMELETTE

Ingredients:

(Makes one large 12"-14" omelette, or two smaller servings)

1/3 cup chickpea flour
1 flax egg (1 tbsp milled flax seed, 1/4 cup warm water)
1 tbsp nutritional yeast
1/2 tsp baking powder
1/4 tsp salt
1/4 tsp garlic powder
1/8 tsp turmeric
1/8 tsp black salt (gives egg flavour)
dash cayenne pepper
1/2 cup water
1/2 cup chopped veggies (scallions, fresh tomato, spinach—whatever sounds good!)

Organic first cold pressed olive oil non-stick cooking spray

Directions:

1. Mix your flax egg and let sit for 5 minutes.
2. Mix all dry ingredients together in a bowl or measuring cup
3. Mix all remaining ingredients together in your bowl
4. If your mix isn't a pancake-like consistency, slowly add more water.
5. Heat a large oiled pan over medium high heat. When ready, pour your mix onto the pan and spread it thinly evenly over your pan. Cover the pan with a lid and cook until the top is "set."
6. Flip the omelette and cook for another couple minutes before it's done.

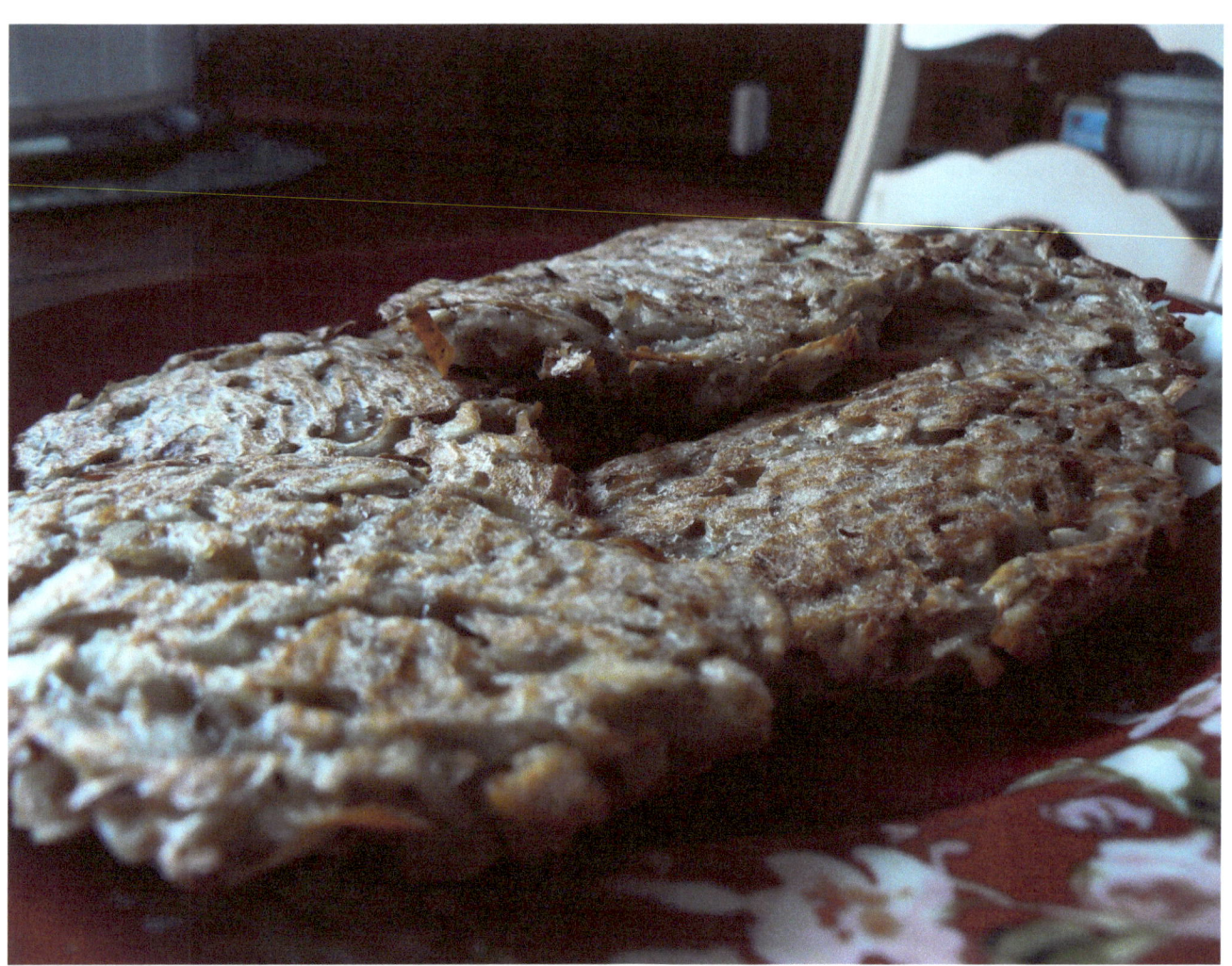

HASH BROWNS

Ingredients:

2 large potatoes, grated
1 small onion
1 teaspoon flax seed powder, mixed with ¼ cup water
¼ cup whole wheat flour
salt and pepper to taste

Parchment paper

Directions:

1. Preheat oven to 375 degrees.

2. Mix all ingredients together well. Should be "pasty" enough to hold together when potato patties are formed.

3. Using hands to shape the patties, make about six and place on parchment paper.

4. Bake 10 minutes on each side (or until bottoms are crisp before turning).

CREATE YOUR OWN RECIPES
UnCommon Substitutions

Egg:
Mix together 1 tsp of flaxseed powder with ¼ cup water for each egg to be replaced.

Milk:
Use Pure, Unsweetened Almond Milk
or Coconut Milk

Oil/Butter or Shortening:

For Baking:
Use applesauce or mashed or pureed fruit in equal quantity

For sauteing:
Saute in water, vegetable broth or wine, instead of oil—usually ½ cup is sufficient to replace oil, but add more as needed.

Sugar:
Agave (sweeter than sugar, so use .75 as a multiplier when figuring how much is enough)

White Flour:
Whole wheat flour in equal quantity.

For home-baked breads, 100% organic whole wheat **bread** flour is available from Great River. You can buy it from www.tropicaltraditions.com

*Open an account on their website and you'll get FREE SHIPPING sales periodically—I wait for these and buy in quantity because sometimes the shipping charges can add up to more than the product total!

***TIPS:

Parchment paper is the key to creating "crispness" to food—line cookie sheet with it and bake in oven, instead of frying. Works great for hash browns, homemade felafels, and just about anything you'd love a little crunchy. You won't miss the oil!

To bring out the flavor and texture of powdered spices —when sauteing, add spices to food and liquid and let all the liquid evaporate. Stir for a minute to coat food, before adding additional liquid for cooking.